I0411495

THE QUIET DIET

*Losing Weight and Live Healthy
While Dieting Secretly*

Table of Contents

The trademarks that are used are without any consent, and the publication of the trademark is without permission or backing by the trademark owner. All trademarks and brands within this book are for clarifying purposes only and are the owned by the owners themselves, not affiliated with this document.

Chapter 1

What is a Healthy Diet?

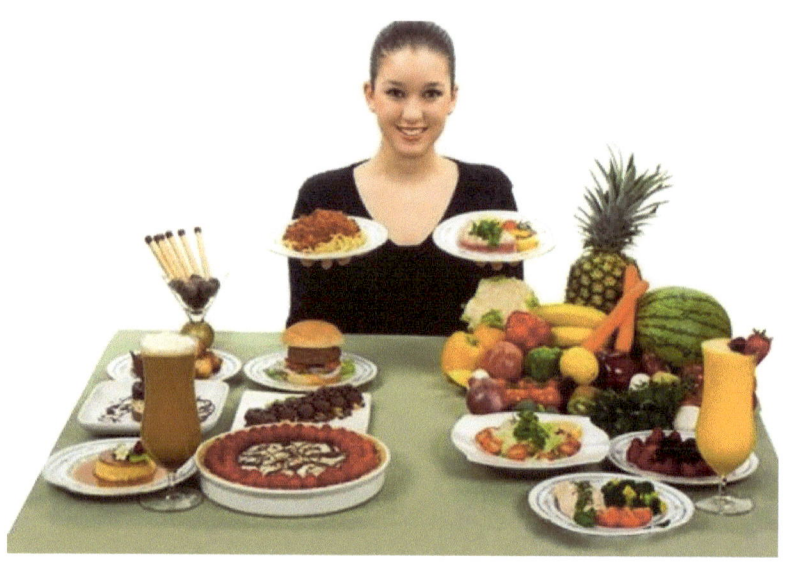

Diet is a prescribed selection of healthy foods and drinks in order to maintain fitness level and lose weight. A healthy diet helps in maintaining all body systems either voluntary or involuntary by generating sufficient energy for the proper functioning. Our digestive system digests food by breaking down macro-nutrients into micro-nutrients and these micro nutrients are now easily assimilated into blood and then supplied to throughout the body where these nutrients generate energy through combustion in the presence of oxygen.

A healthy diet that mainly contains all necessary and important nutrients helps in balancing energy level in our body, but on the other hand the unhealthy diet or a diet that contains insufficient amount of nutrient generally causes low energy level that leads to low rate of metabolism and this kind of diet does not burn extra calories and these untreated calories are the major cause of fat storage in within our body in the form of adipose tissues. These adipose tissues or fat tissues are lack of blood vessels and do not require much energy that's why fat muscles decrease the rate of metabolism.

Contrary to that, muscle tissues that contain sufficient supply of blood vessels require much energy for proper functioning and for this our body generates more energy through increased rate of metabolism. According to the authenticated medical research, a body that contains increased number of muscle mass results in decreased number body fat. A balanced diet provides sufficient energy required for the production of muscle tissue. The energy generated through the combustion of foods also beneficial for over-all physical health such as proper digestion, increased rate of metabolism, proper removal of toxic materials, blood circulation, and respiration and reproduction system.

How Much We Need to Eat

Our need for eat is dependent on different factors such as body temperature, hunger disorder, gastrointestinal tract disorder, bad eating habits, unhealthy foods and nutritional deficiency or malnutrition and physiological activities. Several studies on two different groups of people with less and much physical activities, have shown that the people with more physical activities require more food to eat than the people who involve in less physical activities due to increased rate of metabolism (catabolic reactions: the reactions that break down macro molecules into micro molecules and release energy). Much physical activities require more energy in order to repair or regenerate muscle tissues that breakdown during intense workouts or routine hard works and this required amount of energy is produced by breaking down the food. Only healthy foods give your body a best fuel for better performance. The consumption of food increases with the increase in physical activities in a healthy way.

The Best Way of Eating

The best way of eating is to eat like our body is designed to eat food. I have a plan that you never heard before in your life. Divide your eating strategy in three parts;

- First for the water

- Second for food

- Third for hunger

Explanation

The first part of your healthy meal says that always reserve enormous space in your stomach for water that means drink 1 to 2 glasses of water one hour before your meal in order to make better your digestion and also for stomach health. The second part of eating strategy says that eat healthy foods that are stomach friendly and the last part of the eating strategy says that we need to be sparing in diet and let one third part of stomach for itself for breathing by eating less than your hunger. These habits surely improve your stomach health and digestion as well. The better digestion provides much energy and makes absorption of nutrients better and thus it plays an important role in proper growth and maintenance.

What Type of Diet is the Healthy Diet

The diet includes all necessary and right nutrients such as right type of carbohydrates, protein, fats, minerals and Vitamins. Whole grains, healthy proteins, fats, fresh fruit and vegetables contain healthy carbohydrates and dietary fibers along with minerals and Vitamins that improve our physiological abilities by providing life energy. These vital nutrients not only help in generating energy but also improve our immune system. The diet that contains all natural nutrients (a diet free of refined and processed foods) is the healthy diet that really works.

Diet Constituents

Mainly, our diet contains Vitamins, minerals, carbohydrates, proteins and fats along with water. As described above, these constituents are necessary for the proper functioning of all body systems.

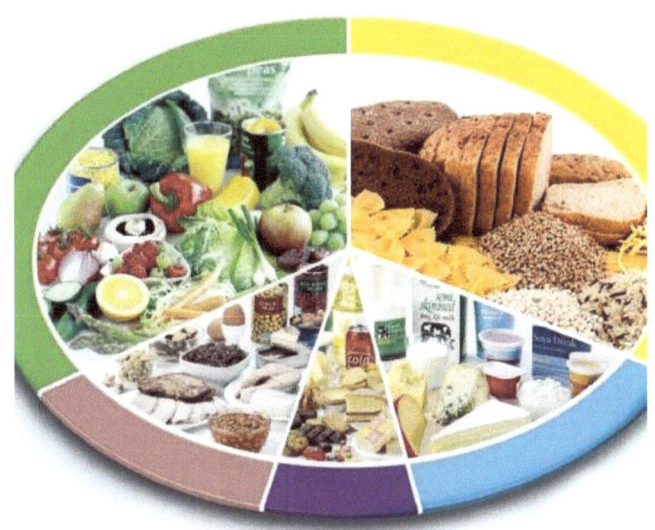

Here are some nutrients that help our body in different ways;

- Right carbohydrates

- Minerals

- Vitamins

- Proteins

- Right fats

- Dietary fibers

Right Carbohydrates

Carbohydrates are the primary source of energy production in our body or the best fuel for our body. According to the majority of the health experts, we should fulfill half of our daily need (nearly 50% of daily need) of calories from carbohydrates. Carbohydrates are found in different foods such as fruits, vegetables, grains and dried beans etc. Our digestive system is a natural system that can digest all natural foods well. Unnatural foods (or the foods not in accordance with nature) cannot be digested in natural way and cannot meet the body needs. All refined and processed carbohydrates are called bad carbohydrates and are hazardous to health.

These bad carbs are digested quickly as compared to natural process of digestion of natural carbs. These quickly digestible carbs can cause several health issues such as digestive problems, excessive production of toxic materials, fast fat storage, type 2 diabetes, hunger disorders and cardiovascular health problems, because these quickly digestible carbs results in sudden increase in glucose and insulin levels. These abnormally increased levels of glucose and insulin badly affect our metabolism.

Avoid or minimize all refined carbs and switch to healthy or complex carbs found naturally in foods high in dietary fibers. The capability of being converted into absorbable condition in the alimentary canal becomes slower than refined carbs and thus this slow process gives you steady blood sugar level. You should consume non starchy fresh fruits and vegetables that are low in glycemic index.

Minerals

Minerals are the important part of our diet that that prevent chronic diseases being important part of our bones and muscle mass. Though minerals are required by our body in a little amount, but we cannot ignore their importance. Minerals in humans, plays their character as electrolytes and as structural and functional elements as well. Minerals can be divided into two groups;

1. Quantity Elements (macro minerals)

2. Essential trace elements (micro minerals)

Macro Minerals

Quantity elements are also called major or macro-minerals and are required the greater amount as compared to micro-minerals or essential trace minerals. Here are some macro-minerals or major minerals;

- Chloride: an important part of sodium chloride (table salt) is important for proper fluid balance in our body and muscle contraction. Table salt and all processed foods are the major sources of chloride.

- Calcium: strengthens teeth and bones. An adequate intake of Calcium through healthy diet, prevents cardiovascular diseases, lowers fat storage within our body and reduces the risks of colon cancer and breast cancer. Dairy products, legumes, a certain type of fish and soy milk are the sources of calcium.

- Phosphorus: phosphorus is important for bone mass. It is also important for acid base balance in our body. Phosphorus determines how our body uses carbs and fat molecules. Phosphorus is also needed for the storage of energy in our body as adenosine tri-phosphate (ATP). It normalizes heartbeat by improving muscle contraction and also important for nerve signaling. Dairy products and proteins are the major source of phosphorus.

- Potassium: potassium is beneficial in blood pressure regulation. It offsets blood pressure raising influences of sodium. The deficiency of potassium may increases the risk of heart diseases and high blood pressure. The major source of potassium is fruits and vegetables.

- Magnesium: it is beneficial for our cells as it causes cellular communication with each other and also makes our healthy and strong by providing energy to our cells for the proper functioning. Magnesium precludes insulin resistance. The major source of magnesium is brown rice, molasses, nuts and seeds, seafood and leafy green vegetables.

- Sulfur: sulfur is found in eggs, meat, fish and poultry. Being a part of our body protein it is an essential for the concentration of muscle and skin protein. Sulfur is necessary for the carbohydrate metabolism, because it is needed for insulin production. Sulfur helps our cells from suffocation caused by the toxins by detoxifying cells.

Micro Minerals

Zinc, Iron, iodine, selenium, copper, manganese, fluoride, chromium and molybdenum etc are the micro minerals and are needed in relatively less amount by our body. Some of the micro minerals are vital for our health like Iron.

Iron is responsible for clear thinking and sufficient supply of oxygen throughout the body for breathing and the combustion of food. Iron is also important for blood protein haemoglobin (a hemoprotein composed of globin and heme that gives red blood cells their characteristic color; function primarily to transport oxygen from the lungs to the body tissues).

Vitamins

Vitamins are the organic chemical substances that organisms require in small or limited amount in order to grow and develop normally. These substances are of different types and can be categorized in two different categories;

1. Fat Soluble

2. Water Soluble

Fat soluble

Vitamin A, D, E and K are fat soluble Vitamins and are absorbed in fat globules. These Vitamins will not be lost event when cooked the foods that contain these fat soluble Vitamins. These vitamins are found in dairy products, liver, oily fish, vegetable oil and salmon.

Water soluble Vitamins

Whereas Vitamin C and B are water soluble and are known as naturally water soluble. Water soluble vitamins do not store within our body and thus these vitamins must be replaced daily. Contrary to fat soluble vitamins, water soluble vitamins are destroyed during cooking, preparing and storing foods containing water soluble vitamins. All citrus fruits contain vitamin C and meat, eggs, fish, legumes, vegetables, cereal grains and milk are the source of vitamin B. vitamin B is known as b-complex group due to the different types of Vitamin B such as B1 (thiamine), B2 (riboflavin), B3 (niacin), B5 (pantothenic acid), B6, B7 (biotin), B12 and Folic acid.

Proteins

Proteins are the complex molecules that contain one or more long chains of amino acids. Protein molecules are also called macro-molecules and are responsible for the development and growth of muscles tissues. Muscle tissues made up of protein molecules and contain a large number of blood vessels and the highest content of mitochondria (an organelle containing enzymes responsible for producing energy) of any tissue in the body and thus these tissues generate more energy by providing ATP (a nucleotide derived from adenosine that occurs in muscle tissue; the major source of energy for cellular reactions). Muscle tissues are also responsible for the movement of all body organs either voluntary or involuntary and responsible for locomotion as well. So, protein is the important part of our body's total mass and we need to add protein rich foods in our diet in order to maintain an optimal health.

Lean protein or lean meat is considered healthy for your heart health and cardiovascular system. So, add lean protein in your healthy diet in order to attain a life without health issues and for strong and healthy muscles.

The Right Fat

Fat is a necessary part of our body, as these molecules build adipose tissue and an adequate amount of adipose tissues cushioning our internal body organs and also function like insulator. But, the amount more than adequate can be hazardous, because an excess of adipose tissues can lead to numerous health issues such as low energy level, diabetes, poor digestion or absorption and excess weight gain.

All types of heart friendly fats are the right fats. According to the majority of health experts, all unsaturated (mono-unsaturated and poly-unsaturated) fat are heart friendly and are good for our health. The sources of good fats are;

- Walnuts

- Olives

- Canola or rapeseeds (canola oil or rapeseed oil)

- Omega 3 fatty acid found in walnut and salmon

- Avocados

- Nuts: peanut and almonds etc

Dietary Fibers

Dietary fibers are the indigestible part of our diet that found in plant matter (plant cell walls). Dietary fiber is also known as roughage. Mainly, there are two types of dietary fibers in accordance with their solubility in water during digestion in our stomach;

1. Soluble dietary fibers

2. Insoluble dietary fibers

Dietary fibers improve absorption of nutrients by our gastrointestinal tract and reduce appetite that causes weight loss in a healthy way. The soluble dietary fibers make a jelly like structure called gelatin that slows the movement of digested food through our gastrointestinal tract and thus it improves absorption of nutrients found in food we eat. Soluble dietary fibers are physiological active byproducts and are fermented in our colon into gases.

Insoluble dietary fibers do not dissolve in water, but these insoluble dietary fibers are fermented in large intestine. Being insoluble in water, insoluble dietary fibers give a bulky effect on eating foods high in fibers such as fresh fruits and vegetables. Insoluble dietary fibers regulate water level, control appetite and make defecation easy along with removing toxic material from gastrointestinal tract.

Chapter 2

Factors Affecting Weight Gain

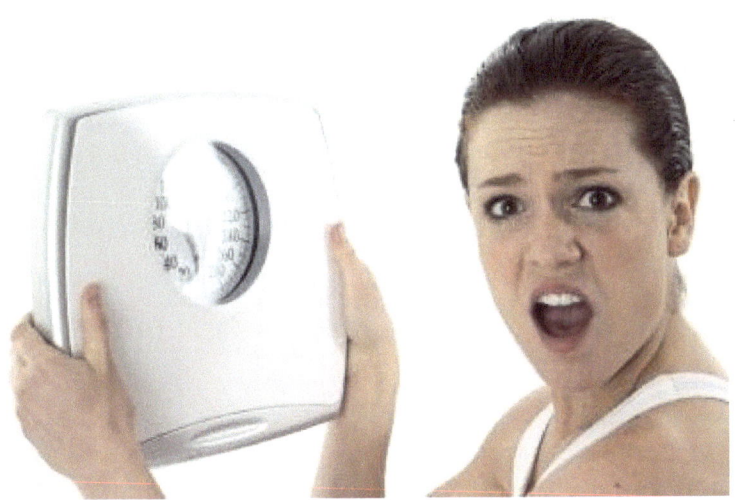

There are several factors that affect our weight badly such as bad eating habits, junk foods, friends addicted to bad foods and bad eating stuff having negative and discouraging nature and especially less mental power or self confidence that directly controls our hormonal system and actions.

Bad eating habit disturbs our digestive system by eating more than our hunger and again and again without feeling hunger. Bad eating habits are caused by bad foods like junk foods. These junk foods are good in taste, but high in calories and also lack of nutrients. Sometimes we fail to maintain our health by adopting natural ways of being healthy due to the people in our surroundings or in our circle that discourage us when we aim to lose weight. Once you have told your friends that you are following a certain diet plan along with an effective exercise plan, then they want to see the change after each passing day and if they don't they discourage you about your diet and exercise plan so, you need to do this secretly or quietly. All we can do is to keep our healthy lifestyle plan secret for quite some time and keep practicing some secret or home base exercises and keep following secret diets such as the quiet diet or the silent diet.

Self confidence and self esteem are the major factors that affect our health and habits. Our increasing weight day by day and discouraging friends make us less confidence. Make your mind and do it with determination if you really want to achieve something you fear most. If you are surrounded by some discouraging people that have negative and criticizing thinking, then you should keep this saying in your mind "**don't worry about those who talk behind your back. They are behind you for a reason.**" It is the only way you can achieve what you want or you deserve for. Just do what you actually need; don't care what the people say. These are some ideas and motivational suggestions that develop self esteem and self confidence and also help you to stick to your aim of losing weigh while following the silent diet.

If you have made a plan of losing weight and you are strictly following it, but suddenly you are discouraged by someone, then you only need to change the plan not the goal. This will encourages you and develops self esteem that results in fast weight loss in quicker short time.

Chapter 3

What is the Quiet Diet

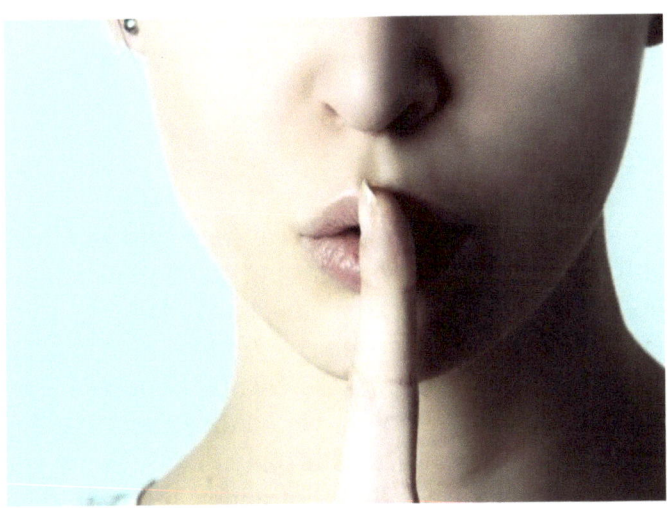

The Quiet diet provides you or facilitates you with such an environment in which you can achieve your desired weight and fitness level and also instill a power of firm determination secretly or without showing it to your friends and other people around you. The quiet diet allows you to choose right foods for you quietly and keeps you natural and healthy without losing self confidence. Decide your foods, their time and amount that you need to eat each time in order to attain a body free of unnecessary fat and physiological health issues. The quiet diet is not involved some specific foods; in fact it is involved healthy eating habits and right types of foods that are produced by the nature for our body. Decreasing caloric intake and increasing physiological activities will surely affect your weigh by shedding some pounds and reducing the size around your belly. Mainly, the quiet diet involves foods that are really affecting and are thoughtful good choices. The quiet diet instills the spirit of self motivation and teaches us "Go over, go under, go around, or go through, but never give up."

Your friends usually dislike your eating style and often feel embarrassed while seeing you skipping modern unhealthy foods and switching to the natural foods. This is the only way you are discouraged by your friends and the people around you and you have to follow your healthy plan secretly or silently.

No, Doesn't Always Mean No

The quiet diet doesn't allow you to eat high calorie foods, but this prohibition or inhibition is not permanent. When you have prepared yourself for intense physical activities, then your body needs more energy in order to rebuild or strengthen muscle tissues and for the peak performance of all physiological functions. And restricted diet plans are then not enough to generate energy for our daily needs. There is something need to follow a diet that generates energy more than restricted diet. And this time you can eat your favorite foods but still under control. You can have your favorite foods that are moderate in calories, but are high in nutritional value.

Role of the Parents in Losing Weight

Parents can play their central role in losing the weight of their adolescent by encouraging them to eat good foods and making them realize with the importance of healthy eating habits and healthy foods. They can make them habitual of healthy foods silently or quietly in order to maintain an optimal fitness by providing them with healthy foods and keeping them away from unhealthy foods that contain less amount of nutrient along with high calories and processed or refined ingredients.

What Should you Do

In order to lose weight you need to do something by yourself. You have to be strong enough to stick to the selection of healthy foods and home base secret exercises. Adopt good eating habits that lead you to the path of extreme fitness. There is no need to do immoral things like lying to your friends and family members about your healthy eating. Become straight forward person and tell them I am just seeking good health and trying to improve my fitness level, because for the few months I am feeling bad health conditions. And if you can't do this just stay silent and eat more slowly and chew your food by taking enough time. This act will save you from over eating the food you want to avoid due to its negative health effects.

Here are some secret tips for healthy eating and attaining optimal fitness while enjoying all blessings of God Almighty;

- Eat slowly, because our stomach signals after being full. Slow eating is the best strategy of losing weight and maintaining good health. Eating slower improves digestion along with good absorption of vital nutrients.

- Eat in three parts in order to sustain life energy and its inner powers. Divide your stomach in three different parts such as one for water, second for food and third for breathing. This means that we should drink one or two glasses of water at least one hour before your meal and eat less than your hunger while keeping some empty space in your stomach for the sake of better digestion and then absorption. This is the secret weapon you can use quietly or without getting loud.

- Hydrate your body in order to normalize all chemical activities within your body. Water provides a necessary medium for the occurrence of all chemical reactions and reduces or normalizes our hunger. An adequate amount of water in our body improves all internal physiological systems such as excretory system, digestive system, auto detox system, blood circulation system and lymphatic system etc. These improves systems enhance physiological abilities and regulate physical energy level. The increased rate of energy level is due to the increased rate of metabolism that results in weight loss in quicker short time.

- Minimize the use of refined sugar and simple sugar as low as you can if you really want to stop gaining weight day by day. You can have tea or coffee with low sugar and switch to complex sugars in place of simple and refined sugars. Although sometimes simple sugar works much better, but not always. All fresh and non starchy fruits and vegetables contain healthy and complex carbohydrates (complex sugars) that are digested more slowly as compared to simple sugars. Simple sugar may lead to imbalance in our blood sugar level and digests quickly. Contrary to that complex sugar digests slowly due to the presence fibers. Complex sugars are also rich with health promoting vitamins and some minerals. So, you need to minimize the use of jams, jellies and all fruit drinks and soft drinks, because these products are high in refined sugar and low in nutritional value.

- Prepare your snacks by your own at home. Boiled beans (with salad and oranges or its alternative such as lemons) and turkey salad (smokes or grilled turkey with salad of high fiber vegetables and leafy green vegetables garnished with almonds or walnuts and black pepper to taste) are prepared at home with ease and comfort.

- Replace refined spices with crushed black pepper (crushed with hands), because black pepper and non refined spices speed up your metabolism and also instill the spirit of doing healthy activities with zeal and excitement. Black pepper contains sufficient amount of antioxidants and have antibacterial effects.

- Switch your processed foods with raw foods, because on cooking several vital enzymes and some of the Vitamins are destroyed and the quality of food is also affected.

- Replace beverages with green tea (lemon, ginger, mint and raw honey) that contains an enormous amount of antioxidants and metabolism booster factors that cause weight loss.

- Reduce stress and anxiety by

- Be wise in parties and events where you have to go unwillingly by adopting wise eating and drinking styles such as you can eat more slowly, by chewing your food or stuff you feel unhealthy and hazardous to your health for much time (by doing this you can eat less food for more time), by drinking too little beverages and alcoholic drinks (better to avoid). Don't feel stress from the foods you don't like due to their negative health effects.

- Do not skip foods as this can lead to nutrition deficiency and can cause several health issues caused by the deficiency of vital nutrients.

Self Motivation

Self motivation is the power of self esteem and self confidence that urges us to do the things we fear most. Self-motivation keeps us on track and does not allow us to leave our goals in spite of thousands of hurdles. Keep motivating yourself by sticking on your plan is the key to achieve optimal fitness and a healthy lifestyle. You can motivate yourself by setting realistic goals, by hanging your favorite outfits on the place you use frequently and by keeping a specific and amazing personality in your mind and challenge to defeat him.

Motivate yourself by taking the challenge that your bad foods and bad eating habits have laid ad your feet.

Change your Today for Better Tomorrow

Think that "you have to change your today for a better tomorrow", because life can seem ungrateful and not always kind. Not today, but after certain duration this time will never be the same and can be hurtful or unfair. If you are trying to change your tomorrow, then one day it can be fair and not hurtful. By trying hard or doing the things good for you, will surely put the beauty in the things you really want to change and beautify. You are offered by your life with its ups and downs, now it is up to you what you choose.

Always choose healthy foods while you are in a party or event with your friends and satisfy yourself with these health foods instead of processed unhealthy foods.

Chapter 4

Easy At-Home Exercises to Lose Weight and Stay Fit

Exercises are the physiological activities which are performed in order to increase physical abilities and to enhance physiological systems that sustain life quality. Exercises are also performed along with healthy diet plan for losing weight in quicker short time in a healthy way. Our body is designed to perform several activities which increase the stability and the range of motion of the different body organs. You can improve your physiological abilities and can achieve peak performance by doing some certain movements designed by certified fitness trainer and physicians.

All physical activities or exercises help in promoting our metabolic health and thus these activities maintain optimal fitness level and healthy muscles by removing extra body fats in quicker short time without leaving any side effect. Exercising regularly is the key to change your lifestyle and to enjoy all your important events you were striving for.

When you are surrounded with some negative or discouraging people that always discourage you from joining a gym and a fitness club by saying that "are you fat or do you really need exercise?", then it is really difficult to fulfill your dream of well shaped body. These all difficulties can be changed to easy ones with firm determination and constantly hard working. The only solution is to practice some home based exercises in order to keep your fitness plan secret from your friends and all the people in your circle.

Losing weight is not as easy as the majority of the people say and is not as difficult as it looks like. Losing and maintaining weight is a system of effective exercises which improve all body muscles and increase our metabolic rate by improving heart beat rate and cardiovascular system. Ruining can improve cardiovascular system and metabolism along with strong legs, but you cannot shape your whole body muscles only running routinely. So, I would like to suggest you a variety of exercise for improving overall muscles which can be practiced at home secretly without joining a gym or a fitness club.

Here are some exercises that will surely help you to maintain a good health without joining a gym or a fitness club;

- A proper warm up

- Pushups (ground and parallel bar pushups)

- Pull-ups

- Squats and other home based exercises for thighs

- Ab workouts

- Shin workouts

- Yoga exercises for inner strength and for gaining life energy

- Some most important and effective stretching exercises

- Metabolism boosting workouts

A Proper Warm up

Warm is generally done before practicing routine exercises in order to prevent muscular injury or muscle pull. A proper warm up not only prevents muscle injury but also increase performance.

Running or low pace jogging for 8 to 10 minutes is the best warm up.

Pushups

Pushups are the generally performed for attaining strong arm and chest muscles. There are several different ways of performing pushups to strengthen different muscles such as forearms, triceps, shoulders and chest muscles. I will suggest you two ways of performing pushups that can be easily performed at your home or office.

Ground Pushups (for chest)

Ground pushups are generally performed manually and usually on the ground and strengthen our arms and chest along with upper back muscles. Here are some tips for performing correctly;

- Down on the ground while supporting your body with your hands on the ground in such a way that your chest should be at a height equal to the distance of your arm's length

- Place your hands 4 to 5 inches wider than your shoulders width in order to perform pushups properly

- Close your both feet together in order to put your maximum weight on your chest muscles

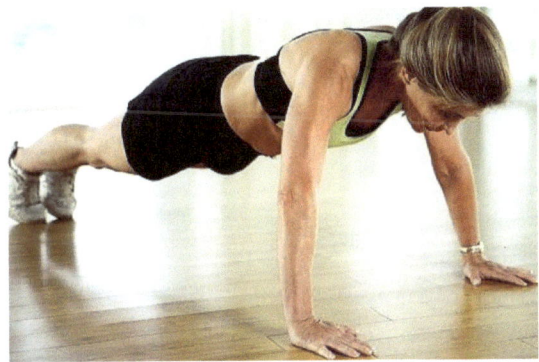

- Keep your hand straight and parallel to each other while keeping your palms downwards

- Now, move your chest downwards while bending your elbows towards your feet and try to touch your chest to the ground or closest to the ground and then move to the starting point

- Do 10 t0 15 times and repeat this workout for 5 to 6 times

Variations

Three variations can be made in order to increases intensity.

1. By placing your hands much greater than your shoulder width

2. By placing your hands less than your shoulder width

3. By using an incline surface or wearing a weight bag on your back for increasing intensity of pushups

Pushups for Arms

Pushups can be practiced for strengthening your arm muscles. Here are some tips that will help you in strengthening your arm muscles without joining a gym;

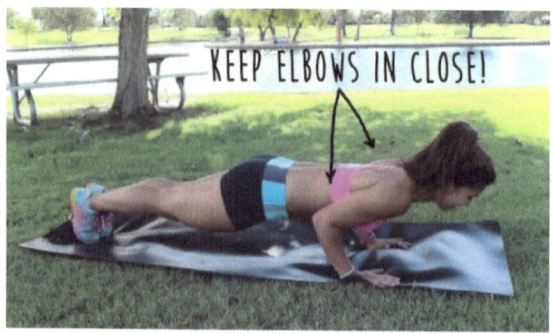

- Get in pushup position while closing your elbows to your side belly on both sides

- Keep your hands parallel to each other and your palms should be downwards

- Slightly bend your elbows towards your feet and do pushups in slow pace

- Do 10 t0 15 pushups and repeat this workout for 4 to 5 times

Triangular Pushups

Doing pushups while making triangle with both your hands, is an effective workout for your triceps and your arms. It can be performed easily by newbie or a starter.

- Get it pushups position while opening your hands a little less than your shoulder width

- Touch your both elbows to your side belly (each side)

- Make a triangle with both your hands in such a way that touch your both thumbs with each other and index fingers (the finger next to the thumb) with each other

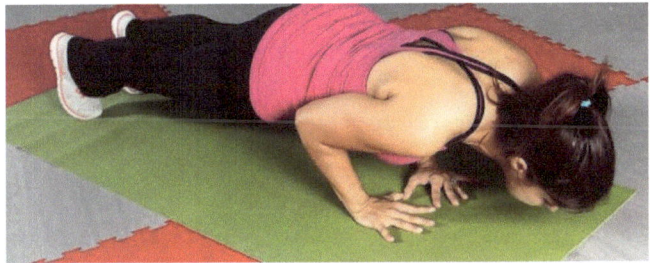

- Now do your pushups in slow pace for at least 10 to 15 times

- Repeat this exercise for 5 to 6 time

Pushups for Beginners

The beginners can do pushups from their knees instead of feet. Pushups on knees are easy to do. After a week try to do full pushups in order to achieve expected results.

If you have some health issues and can't do pushups even on knees, then you can hold your pushups position only without doing pushups in order to strengthen your core muscles that are involved in pushups.

Pushups or Dips on Parallel Bar

Pushup on parallel bar is an effective workout that not only shapes your upper body but also strengthens your core. This workout is an advanced form of pushups and dips. There are several physical activities that can be performed on parallel bar, but here we will learn only upper body workout especially for chest and arm muscles.

- Stand before a parallel bar (the bars height should be less than your chest or equal to your chest) and hold the bars with your hands and lift your whole body while supporting your body with your hands

- Fold your legs from knees while crossing over your lower legs(shins) with each other

- Now, slowly move down your body while hanging your folded legs from knees

- Move as down as possible with ease and comfort (don't let your body down below your elbow level, because this will prevent great stress on your shoulder muscles) and then move to starting position

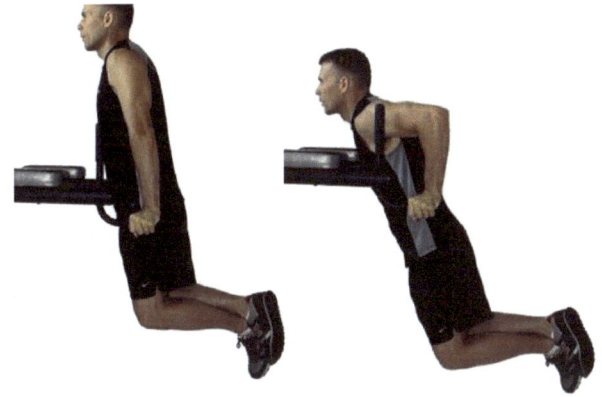

- Do 10 to 15 reps and repeat this workout 4 to 5 times while taking recovery period for 30 seconds or according to your fitness level

- Do not let your body down from you cannot lift it up. Always be careful while practicing on parallel bars neither practice too much on the bars nor do rapid moves in order to prevent muscle injury

Pull-Ups

Pull up is the best workout to test your physical abilities and inner or core strength. Pulling your body in upward direction while lifting your hanging body with your arms only, involves upper body muscles such as upper back/front, biceps, triceps and shoulder muscles. There are different ways of practicing pull ups depending on the muscles involved in this workout;

1. Pull ups for biceps

2. Pull ups for shoulder and chest muscles

Pull ups for Biceps

Here are some tips that will help you in practicing pull ups correctly;

- Hang from a bar while supporting your whole body with your hands (straight)

- Fold your legs and keep your palms towards your face

- Wide your hands a little bit wider than your shoulder width

- Raise or lift your body in upward direction and try to touch your chest or chin to the bar while keeping your whole body straight except your knees

- Do at least 10 to 12 reps and repeat this workout for 4 to 5 times

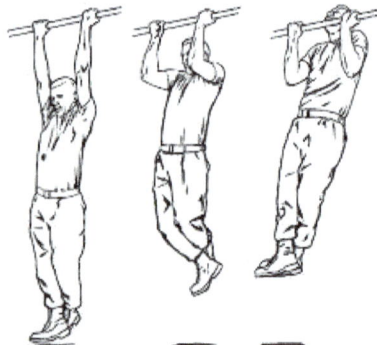

- Variations can be made by wearing a weight bag and holding some weights with your folded shins in order to increase force

- Always do some stretching workouts before and after any exercise in order to increase the range of motion of your body muscles

Squats

Squat training is a type of strength training that improves and trains lower body muscles such as thigh muscles or quadriceps (vastus lateralis, rectus femoris, vastus medialis and vastus intermedius), hips, hamstrings and buttocks. Squat training also improves the physical ability of lower body portion and increases the range of motion of muscles involved in this training.

Squat exercise is performed in different styles depending on different outputs. The main muscles that involve in this workout are quadriceps, gluteus and hamstrings.

How to Perform (beginners)

- Stand in a comfortable environment while wearing easy or comfortable cloths

- Raise your hands in front of you while making 90 degree angle between your chest and arms

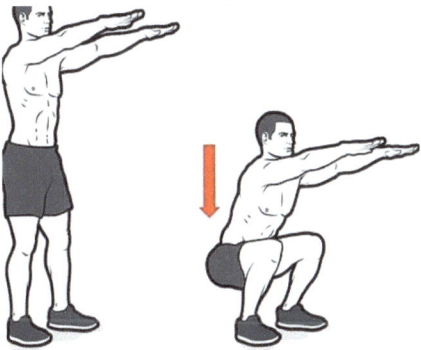

- Open your legs little wider than your shoulder width

- Now, slowly move your body downwards without bending your upper body or keeping your upper body straight

- While moving down do not sit completely, and move upward or starting position

- Be careful while doing your squats and try to keep your back straight in order to prevent back pain and leave this training or reduce your reps if feel pain during your workout

- do 15 to 20 times and repeat this exercise for 3 to 4 times

- Variations can be made after practicing beginner's squat training or improving your core muscle quality. In advanced squat training you can wear a weight bag on your back while practicing squat training at home.

Squats by using Resistance Bands

You can practice squat workouts by using resistance band in order to improve your lower muscle quality and also for shaping them in quicker short time at home. Here are some tips to correctly perform squat training with the help of resistance band;

- Wrap a resistance band over your shoulders in such a way that the both ends of the resistance band should be tied to your feet

- Hold squat position (the down position) it is contrary to the normal squat exercise in which you start your workout from standing straight, but this time you have to start from bending position. Bend your body while making 90 degree angle between your thighs and shin muscles

- Make sure resistance band is neither too tight nor too lose

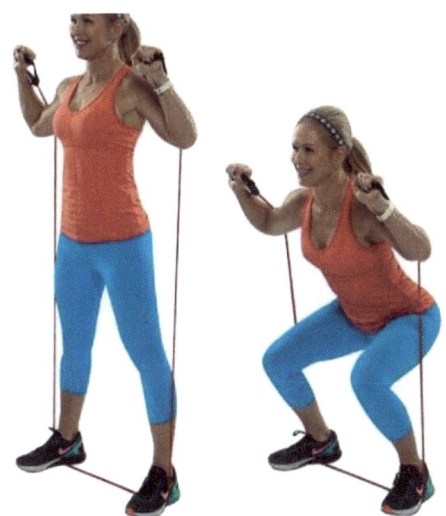

- Now, move upwards and stand straight and them again move down with the force of resistance band

- Do at least 12 to 15 reps and repeat this exercise 3 to 4 times

Ma Bu (The Kun Fu Squat)

Ma Bu stance is generally practiced in Kung Fu trainings for strengthening core muscles of lower body portion. Ma Bu is also practiced for developing self confidence and life quality. It can be practiced without equipments or with equipments.

Here are some tips to perform Ma Bu stance;

- Stand straight and open your legs little bit wider than your shoulder width

- Now move down while making 90 degree angle between your thighs and shins and thighs and belly

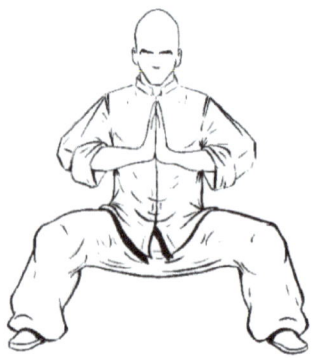

- Hold this position as long as you can bear and after leaving this position take rest for 30 sec to 1 minute and then do it again

- Repeat this workout for 3 to 5 times

Variation can be made by using a resistance band and following the simple steps given below

- Hold Ma Bu position and wrap a resistance band

- Pull resistance band to make it tight too much

- Now, bend to hold Ma Bu position. After bending, resistance band becomes less tight than before, but after bending it still exerts a downwards force that helps you in strengthening your lower body muscles in a few days amazingly

- Hold this position as long as you can bear

- Repeat this exercise for 4 to 5 times

Ab Workouts

Belly shape plays an important role in shining our personality. Our abdomen is a part of our body that stores stubborn adipose tissues in large number. Belly fat is considered more stubborn fat within our body and is most difficult to remove especially after giving birth to a baby or after 30 years age. In the people, who do not care about their health and used to eat unhealthy foods and do less or no physical activities suffer from obesity or excess body fat. The excess body fat not also affect their body shape but also disturb body's internal systems such as excretion, digestion, blood circulation and endocrine systems etc. Excess body fat also cause cardiovascular diseases and deteriorates or degrades mental health along with less confidence.

Here are some belly workouts that can be performed at home or at your office especially for the people who cannot joint a gym or a fitness club just because of their surrounding people who often discourage them to do such kind of physical activities to improve your health;

- Abdominal core strengthening workouts

- Cardiovascular exercises for faster metabolism

- Advanced ab workouts

- Belly workouts by using ab roller

Belly warm up

As described above that warm is necessary for enhancing your performance and to prevent muscular injury or pain. Warm is also beneficial for better blood circulation and energy generation for performing different powerful movements in order to lose fat. So, warm for belly workout is very important and necessary. You can do belly warm by lying down on the exercises mat or some cushioning material and cycling with both your legs while keeping your upper body motionless after jogging or running for 5 to 6 minutes. Running improves heart quality and thus it supplies more blood to your body organs and generate enormous energy for the proper functioning of all physiological systems. Belly warm up allows you to perform abdominal exercises with ease and comfort.

Abdominal Core Strengthening Workouts

Belly is the most important part of our body that represents our fitness level more clearly than others. The majority of the people who want to do some ab workouts, but fails due to weak belly muscles and find it more difficult to shape and usually adopt other methods to reduce belly fat. This is due to the reason that they have weak core and if they improve their core quality, they can burn their belly fat through a proper way of exercising for which our body is designed.

Here are some tips to do abdominal core strengthening exercises;

- Lying down on the exercise mat or a cushioning material like a carpet etc. On your back band your knees while lifting them from ground and your feet on the ground

- Do not close your legs and bend your knees in such a way that there must be a gap between your hamstring and calf making "V" shape of your legs

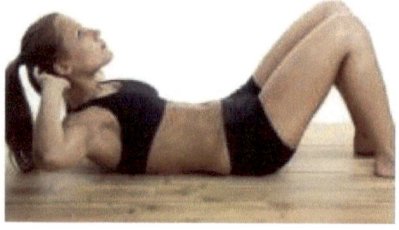

- Now try to raise your chest towards your knees while keeping your knees still or motionless. Raise your body while making "V" shape of your knees and belly and rest your hands on your neck or the back of your head

- Hold this position for 20 to 30 sec or according to your physical health condition

- Release the hold and recover your body for 12 sec and hold this position again

- Do at least 10 to 15 times or greater

- Repeat your workout for 5 to 6 time

Variations

Variations can be made by practicing this exercise in the same position while raising your shins together making 90 degree angle between your shins and hamstrings. This pose will exert more force than previous one and you will get expected results in two to three weeks. To make your crunches more intense do the same hold while holding weights in your hands in front of you and move your hands over your head and then back to your raised knees.

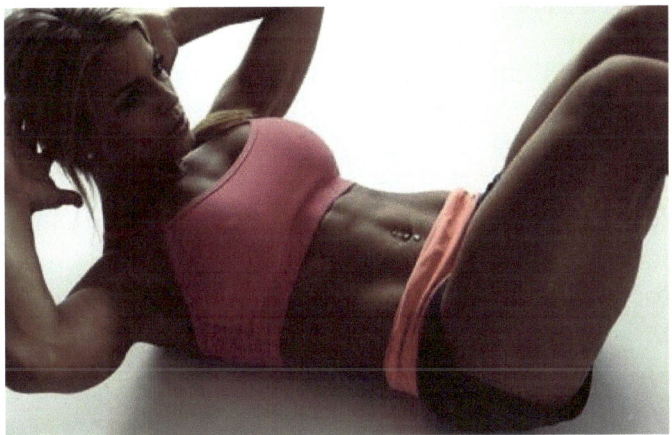

Plank Hold

Plank hold is an effective workout that improves front thigh muscles, abdominal muscles and shoulder muscles. Plank hold can be practiced at anywhere, because it doesn't require any equipment except an exercise mat. Here are some tips that will help you to perform plank hold in an appropriate way;

- Hold pushup position on your forearms instead of hands on a carpeted floor or the exercise mat

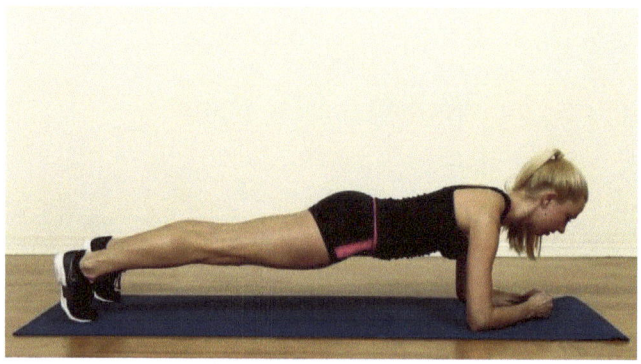

- Raise your abdomen or belly as much as you can without making curve

- Focus on your front belly muscles and hold this position for 20 to 30 seconds

- Do 5 to 6 time and repeat this workout for 4 to 5 times

Variations

Variations can be made by wearing a weigh bag on the upper back of your body. This hold is difficult and should be practiced by the advanced athletes or the people who are used to exercising routinely.

Ab workouts using Ab Roller

An ab roller is an effective tool for your abs, because it can be used anywhere anytime you need to do some physical activities. It is an easy exercise with amazing results and gradually increases intensity.

Rollout for Beginners

- Sit in a comfortable environment on your knees like a cat style while holding an ab roller

- Slowly roll your ab roller or ab wheel in front of you

- Move forward as long from where you can easily pull back your ab wheel

- Pull back ab roller and do this rollout again

- Do at least 15 to 20 reps and repeat this workout for 3 to 4 times

- If you can't do this easily, then sit on your back while opening your both legs in front of you in "V" shape

- Hold an ab roller and place it in front of your crotch

- Start rolling ab roller in forward direction and pull back from your feet

- Do 15 times and repeat this exercise for 3 to 4 times

Rollout for Advance Athlete

Athletes or the people who are used to exercising routinely need more intense workout for the development of new muscles tissues that are stronger than previous ones. After strengthening your core and practicing beginner ab workout you can easily perform full range of ab workout. Here are some tips for practicing intense ab workout;

- On your feet, stand holding your ab roller

- Now, place your ab roller on the ground and hold pushups position

- Now, try to pull back the ab roller towards your feet and then again forward

- You can start this rollout from your feet in forward direction too

- Do at least 12 to 15 times or according to your belly core quality or strength

- Repeat ab workout for 3 times

Variations

Variations can be made by using an inclined plane and rolling ab roller on an inclined surface instead of floor in order to increase intensity and to get expected results in no time.

How to   Remove Belly Fat at Home

Shin workout strengthens your lower body muscles below your knees called shank or shin (the leg between knee and ankle) and improves muscle quality.

Heel Raise

Heel raise is an effective exercise for shin muscles that shapes your shin in a few days and also enhances calf muscle power that improves your jumping ability.

- Do a proper warm up and stretching exercises

- Stand straight while resting your hands on your hips

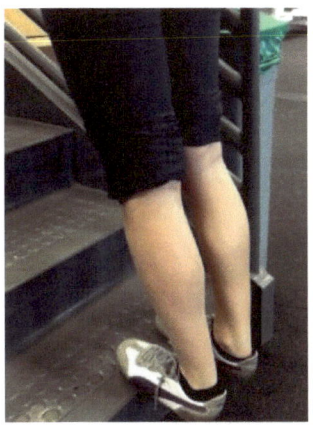

- Open your feet at one hand width in order to balance your body while practicing heel raise workout

- Slowly raise your heels with the help of your toes

- After reaching peak position move downwards and then again upwards and so on

- Do 20 to 30 reps each time and repeat this workout for 3 to 4 times

Variations

Variations can be made by doing this exercise while standing on an inclined surface or by using stairs (stairs are also work like an inclined surface). If you are failed to find an inclined surface around you, then you can make inclined yourself too by supporting a pole or a wall and resting your feet 3 to 4 feet away from the pole or wall. I often used to do this exercise by wearing weight bag or lifting a weight on my shoulders, because it exerts more force on my calf muscles.

Yoga or Meditation

Yoga exercises are generally performed to promote inner strength and for spiritual health.

Yoga exercises are also practiced to promote control of the body and mind through different stances. Here are some yoga techniques that will surely help you to control and to promote core strength of belly;

- Yoga Pilate

- Bow pose

- One hand raised plank

Yoga Pilate

Here are some tips to correctly perform yoga Pilates at home;

- All you have to do that sit in a comfortable environment on the carpeted mat or on the exercise mat

- Concentrate your whole body weight on your hips (while supporting your whole body with your hips on the ground)

- Straight your back and neck while making "V" shape of your legs and belly. First raise your knees and then raise your feet skywards

- Hold this position for at least 15 seconds

- Repeat this exercise for 4 to 5 times

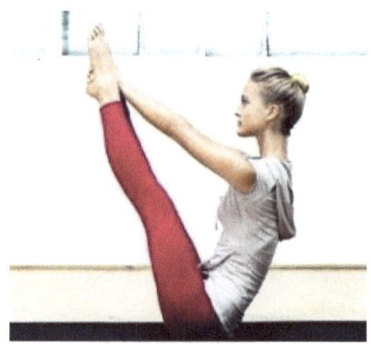

Variations

Variations can be made by bending your knees in front of your parallel to horizon. This variation makes your practice easier than "V" shape pose. If you want to make it more intense, then simply practice "V" shaped pose while raising your both hands skywards.

Bow Pose

Bow pose stretches your belly muscles and increases the range of motion of muscles involved in this practice. This stance also increases the flow of blood through the muscles involved in this position and thus it generates energy for the proper functioning of belly muscles and to regenerate stronger muscles.

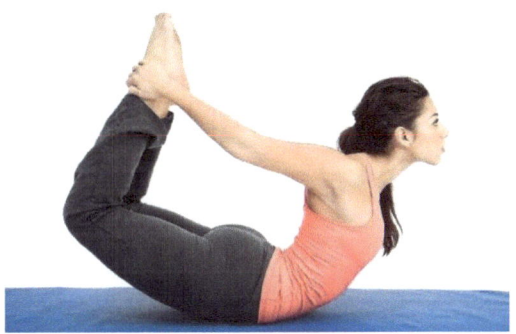

Follow these simple steps for correctly doing bow pose for your belly;

- Lie down your belly on the exercise mat

- Raise your shoulders and legs in upward direction without moving your belly and make a curve. You can easily lift your chest by pressing or holding your feet and pulling them towards upper back of your shoulders

- Avoid stressing excess force on your legs while pulling them in order to prevent back pain

- Hold this position as long as possible (do not hold your position more than 1 minute)

- Release position in case of any pain

- Repeat bow pose for 3 to 4 times

One Hand Raised Plank

One hand raised plank workout allows you to put more stress on your abdominal muscles than other plank workouts and thus it helps in losing belly fat in a few days.

Follow these simple steps in order to perform one arm raised plank workout;

- Hold pushups position on the exercise mat or on the carpeted floor

- Wide your hands one hand wider than your shoulder width

- Raise your one hand sidewise and hold for 10 to 15 sec or according to your fitness level and then move downwards (starting point). Your raised hand's direction should be towards your ear or head

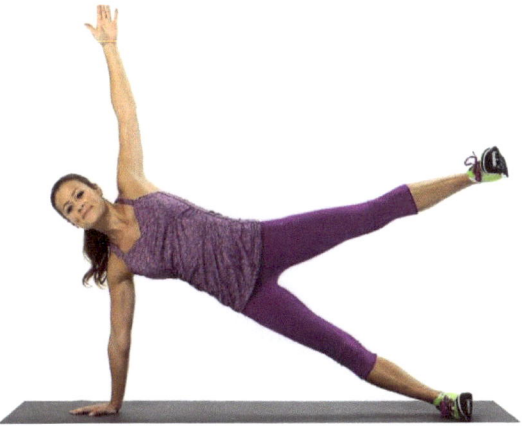

- Recover your belly for 5 to 8 sec and this time raise sidewise your other hand

- Now, release your position and rest for 20 to 30 seconds and then again hold your position and do the same workout

- Repeat this exercise 3 times

Variations

Variations can be made by holding some weights in your raised hands.

- Hold pushups position or stance while holding weights in your hands

- Width of your hands should be the same as that of previous position

- Raise your hand with weight in your hand and hold this position for the same time or according to your physical ability

Repeat 3 to 4 times this whole procedure

Chapter 5

At-home Exercise to Boost Your Metabolism

All biochemical or organic reactions occurring in our body as a whole are called metabolism. Metabolism can be divided into two divisions with respect to their constructive and destructive activities. These two types of metabolism are;

- Catabolism (destructive biochemical reactions: breakdown in living organisms of more complex substances into simpler ones together with release of energy)

- Anabolism (constructive biochemical reactions: the synthesis in living organisms of more complex substances from simpler ones together with the storage of energy)

Metabolism is responsible for the energy generation processes and thus it helps in improving all body organs either voluntary or involuntary. With the age our metabolic rate lowers and affects all physical systems that sustain life quality. There is something need to be done for boosting up the metabolic rate in order to sustain a good health. According to the medical research on metabolism, physical activities performed routinely can increase metabolic rate to a healthy extent.

Cardiovascular exercises are considered a healthy way of boosting metabolism, because it generates energy through aerobic energy generation process. All cardio exercises are powered by aerobic metabolism that generates energy in the presence of sufficient amount of oxygen. Cardio exercises are best way of boosting metabolism in a healthy way. Cardiovascular exercises improve heart efficiency by strengthening cardiac muscles, strengthen respiratory muscles, reduce high blood pressure, increase the amount of red blood cells and thus supply enough oxygen throughout the body.

Cardio workouts can be performed in a variety of ways such as swimming, long distance running, walking, jogging, cycling, rowing and kick boxing.

Swimming is the best cardio exercise that burns fat in quicker short time along with elevated heart rate. You can practice some cardiovascular exercises at home in order to remove fat secretly. You can practice cardio exercises while using stationary bicycle or a treadmill at home. Stair climbing is another cardio exercise that can be performed at home with ease and comfort. Make stairs climbing and running in low pace as your daily routine in order to maintain heart health and to prevent cardiovascular diseases. You can practice it early in the morning at your home or in the park after a proper warm up. After a few days of your starting cardio exercises, you can increase the intensity of your workout in order to achieve optimal fitness level. For example, if you have been practicing stair climbing for a few days, then you can increase your intensity by skipping one stair each time while climbing or you can simply practice stair climbing while wearing a weight bag on your back in order to increase the intensity of your cardio exercise. If you are going to somewhere with your friends who never support you in exercising and because of them you are worried about your exercise, then it's really a big problem and is difficult to manage in such kind of situation. In this situation you can still do your exercises, but this time you have no routine all you can do is to take advantage of opportunity of climbing stairs steep paths, lifting luggage and doing other tasks. These are your secret techniques to avail every opportunity of doing physical activities and burning excess calories.

Stretching Exercises

According to the majority of the physiotherapists and bone & joint specialist, stretching exercises improves joint functioning, increases the range of motion of the muscles and prevent muscular injury or muscle pull during intense workouts.

Stretching exercises are generally performed in order to achieve flexibility, comfortable muscle tone, muscle control and to increase the range of motion of muscles. After getting muscular injury, a physiotherapist suggests stretching exercises as a best remedy to heal muscular injury or to alleviate cramps that is a painful and involuntary muscular contraction. In fact stretching is an inborn behavior that is simply called instinctive behavior that can be seen in others or you can feel in yourself after prolonged sitting, inactivity or sleep. Our body naturally flexes some muscles in order to refresh them or tone them. On the other hand less or no stretching exercises results in arterial stiffness, muscle spasticity, musculotendinous strain and muscle weakness.

Here are some stretching exercises that are necessary to improve your joints and muscles;

Neck Stretch

- Always do dynamic stretches before practicing static stretches in order to do a proper warm up that helps you in performing correct moves and minimizes the possibilities of muscular injury

- stand straight, losing your hands downwards

- open your feet at shoulder width or as much wider as you can balance your body well

- Now, move your neck in downward direction to touch your chin with your chest without moving your whole body and then move back to starting point. After that move your neck in backward direction as back as possible while looking skywards

- Hold both these stretching exercises for 3 seconds

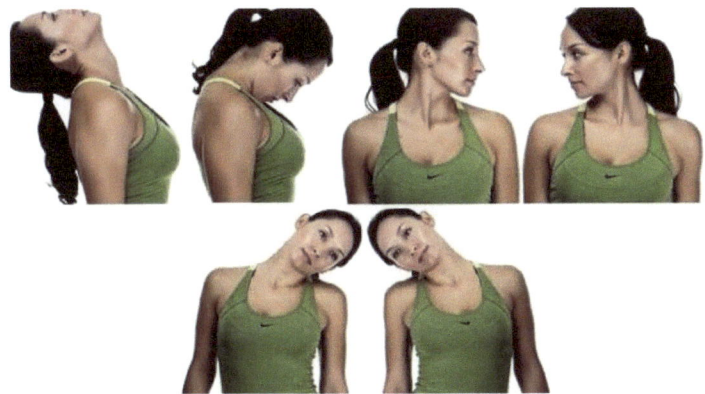

- Take some rest for next move

- Now, move your neck sidewise (left and right in order to touch each shoulder with your ear). Do this exercise in dynamic stretch for warm up

- Hold this stretching exercise for 2 to 3 sec

- Rest for 20 to 30 seconds for recovery

- Now, move your neck sidewise making 360 degree angle with your nose along X-axis while moving your nose towards each shoulder

- Hold this stretch for 2 to 3 sec

- Take rest for some time and then rotate your neck while making as large circle in the sky with your nose as possible. In this stretching exercise move your neck in all possible direction and try to move your muscles in maximum range (your chin should slide over your chest while making the largest circle in the sky with your nose).

- Do this exercise for 8 to 10 seconds

This is the complete warm up and stretching exercise for your neck muscles that incredibly increase the performance of your neck muscles and the range of motion as well.

Stretch for Hamstrings

Hamstrings are the tendons (hamstrings are also termed as muscles) which are contracted by semimembranosus, semitendinosus and biceps: the thigh muscles. Hamstrings are responsible for the knee flexion and hip extension. Flexible hamstrings increase the range of motion of our torso while moving downward. Hamstrings are involved in different body movements such as walking, running, jumping and moving downwards while picking something from ground.

- Do a proper warm up by running or walking for 5 to 10 minutes in cardio style

- Stand straight opening your legs less wider than your shoulders

- Now move your torso or trunk in downward direction in order to touch your toes without bending or opening your knees

- Do not stay at any point try to move all the time during this stretching exercise for better results

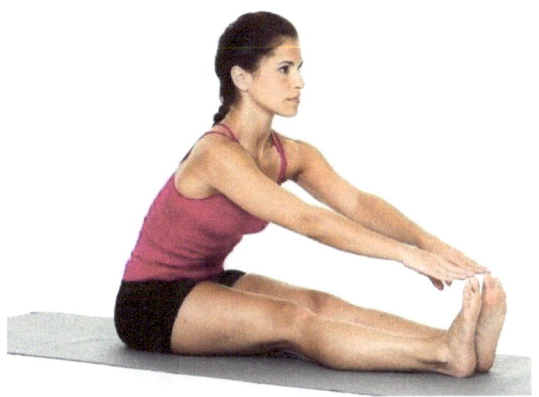

- Do at least 2 minutes or according to your fitness level

- Take some rest for recovery and then sit down and straight your legs while joining both your feet

- Pull your toes towards you while keeping straight your upper body

- Now, try to touch your toes without bending your knees and hold this position for 2 to 3 sec

- Release the position if you feel any pain and massage our thighs with a good oil in order to soften your muscles and for better blood circulation and then do your exercise again.

Variations

Variations can be made by following these simple tips;

- Stand near a bench or bench like fixed support

- Rest or place your one leg on the high back of the bench or a fixed support (the height of the bench or some supporting material should be equal to your belly) and the other leg on the ground

- Now, move your upper body downwards in order to touch your toes on the ground without bending your both knees while touching your right ear to your right leg (bending towards your right side belly)

- Do the same exercise for your left hamstring by changing your leg position from right to left

Elbow Pull

Do a warm up for the shoulder by circling your both arms in clockwise and anticlockwise direction to prevent injury and to perfectly stretch your shoulders. Follow these simple instructions to correctly stretch your shoulder muscles;

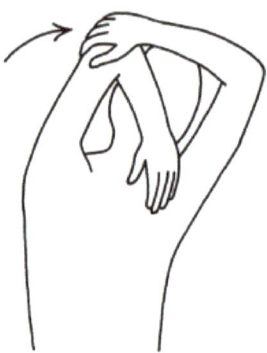

- Stand straight and open your feet at your shoulder width

- Raise your right hand vertically and Hold your left back shoulder with right hand. The direction of your right elbow should be skywards

- Hold your right elbow with left hand in order to pull this elbow for stretching

- Pull your right elbow towards behind your head and move slightly for 5 to 6 times and then hold stretched position for 3 sec

- Repeat this stretch for 4 to 5 times for each shoulder

Variations can be made by changing the position of your elbow from vertical to horizontal.

Side Shoulder Stretch

- Stand straight and raise your right hand in horizontal direction while making right angle between your chest and raised arm

- Move your forearm without moving your elbow and hold your shoulder

- Grip this bent elbow with left hand exactly from the bent joint of elbow and slowly pull your bent elbow across your chest in order to stretch right shoulder muscles

- Hold this stretch for 3 sec, keeping your neck straight

- Repeat this stretch for 5 times for both shoulders

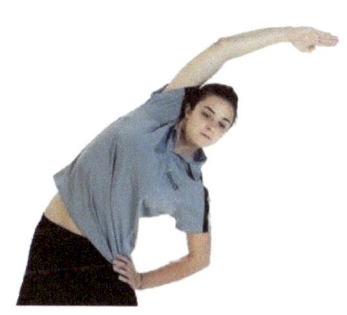

Upper Back Stretch

- Stand straight, interlace your fingers and raise your hands above your head. Turn palms upwards or in skyward direction.

- Move your interlaced hands in backward direction in order to stretch upper back shoulder muscles

- Stretch your shoulders for at least 8 to 10 sec each time

- Repeat this exercise 6 to 8 times

Side Stretch

- Hold upper back stretch position keeping your interlaced hands above Your head

- Move your upper body each side one after the other without moving lower body portion

- First stretch to right side and move as down as possible and hold this stretch for 4 to 5 sec and do this exercise for each side

Chapter 6

How to Handle Social Pressure While Dieting

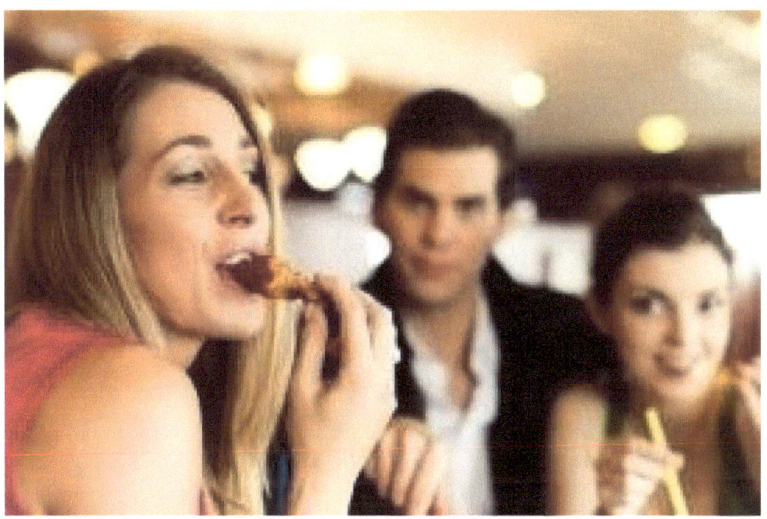

It's hard to follow a healthy diet plan when people close to you are involved. It is more difficult when you're eating out with friends or family.

Eating out is a fun as you enjoy time with friends or family. But whenever you eat out, you usually overdo it. Your family and friends want to entice you with high calorie treats even if they are fully aware you're attempting to drop some weight. This type of pressure from peers is usually annoying, no doubt. These 5 tips will assist you stay focused. You could even motivate them to participate in your cause.

Portion control

Generally, People in America need to have about 2,000 calories every day, and understanding the best way to determine a portion size can assist you achieve that goal. If you are getting pasta, a best suggestion is to have a portion that seems to be almost the size of your closed fist. Same thing goes with the meat.

Eat before you Go

If you understand that you'll be experienced with lots of treats at a get together, it is beneficial to eat something filling just before you go. A healthy salad is an excellent decision due to the fact it's low in calories, but helps make you really feel contented for a couple of hours. Low fat protein sources such as seafood, chicken, and legumes have the similar filling impact. You will believe that it is much simpler to ignore rich foods if your stomach is already full.

Soup and salad

One more method to follow your diet plan would be to order a healthy salad or soup as first. There's some proof to demonstrate that people who eat a soup or a salad just before their meal usually eat less calories for the full meal.

Serve Yourself

You can still follow your healthy and balanced eating ability when eating with other people. Fill up 1 / 2 your plate with fresh fruit or veggies, a 1 / 4 with animal meat or health proteins, and a 1 / 4 with starchy foods. Or you can replace starchy food with some other foods.

If you are unable to make your own plate, there is certainly nothing inappropriate with requesting the server for smaller sized servings. Eventually, although, it could be much better to run away from your diet plan one time than hurt the host by having absolutely nothing more than a handful of nuts.

Share your Diet Details

You really feel good because you began eating much healthier, and obviously you would like to discuss that with other people. But in case your associates are not willing to analyze their dietary habits, forcing them to stay away from foods full of fat and sugar could seem like rubbish.

Be healthy and prove them the effects of healthy eating. As it is said, "Actions speak louder than words."

If you do not wish to be hassled about your eating habits, really don't place your buddies on the place either. Put it off till they show attention in your diet plan. Then calmly discuss the information.

Conclusion

Thank you again for downloading this book!

I hope this book was able to help you to lose weight and live healthy while dieting secretly.

The next step is to remember your healthy eating habits and continue them.

Finally, if you enjoyed this book, please take the time to share your thoughts and post a review on Amazon. It'd be greatly appreciated!

Thank you and best wishes.

www.ingramcontent.com/pod-product-compliance
Lightning Source LLC
Chambersburg PA
CBHW040324010626

45792CB00024B/2115